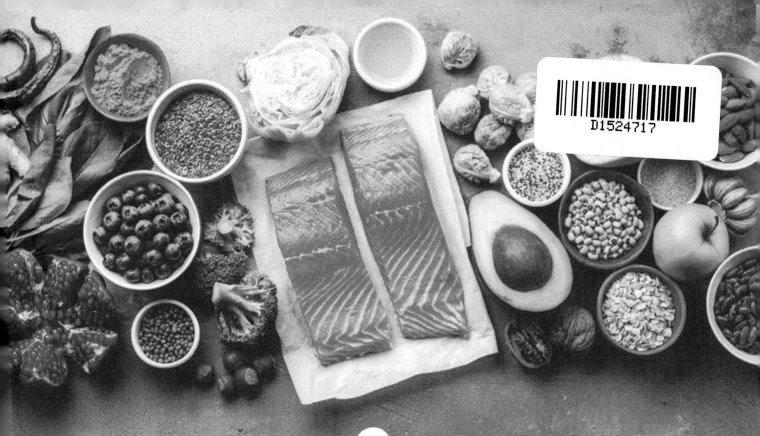

Mindfulness Keto

4 WEEK

KETO DIET PROGRAM

WORKBOOK

Jennifer Stewart

MINDFULNESS KETO
4 WEEK KETO DIET PROGRAM
WORKBOOK

Intro

If you're reading this, then you've decided you're ready to change your health, your looks, and how you feel with the help of my four-week Keto Diet Program. Congratulations! You're here because you're ready to take control and start losing healthy weight.

Before you jump right in, though, you should know that like all life changes, this one is going to be a definite change. It's different, and it's not always easy, but if you stick to it, you'll find that the results are well worth the challenges you face.

So, welcome to the program! This workbook is meant to make the whole diet feel less like a constrictive effort to lose weight, and more like a journey to a whole new, better life.

Oh, and one more thing: I am not a doctor. My Keto diet program is not meant to treat or diagnose any health issues or illnesses. It is a program that I have developed through extensive research and personal experience. While my results have been amazing, you may not experience the same results, as individual results will likely vary.

Before you attempt this diet, or any of the recommended fasting, consult your doctor.

BEFORE YOU START THE KETO DIET

As with all things, the more you know, the more power you will have. The same is true of the Keto diet. There are some things that you need to know before you commit to it.

What is Keto

A ketogenic diet is well known for being a low carb diet. Essentially, when you cut your carbs significantly, your body changes the way it burns fat. Lower carb intake causes the body to produce ketones in the liver. These ketones are used as energy.

When you eat foods that are high in carbs, your body produces glucose and insulin.

- **Glucose** is the easiest molecule for your body to convert and use as energy so it will be chosen over any other energy source.

- **Insulin** is produced to help process the glucose in your bloodstream by carrying it around the body.

Since glucose is being used as a primary energy source, the fats that your body has so carefully stored away are not needed and this causes them to stay in their storage spots (i.e. the thighs). Typically, with a normal, higher carbohydrate diet, the body uses glucose as its main form of energy. By lowering the intake of carbs, the body goes into a state known as ketosis. Being in ketosis puts your body in fat burning mode.

Ketosis is a natural process that the body initiates to help it survive when food intake is low. While in this state, we produce **ketones**, which are made from the breakdown of fats in the liver.

The goal of a properly maintained keto diet is to force your body into this metabolic state, so that it becomes easier for the body to burn excess stored fats. We don't do this through starvation, or drastic reduction of calories, but through dramatically reducing carbohydrates.

By keeping carbohydrates limited and making sure that they come mostly from vegetables, nuts, and dairy, you're going to optimize your nutrition, and help your body go into ketosis. Don't eat any refined carbohydrates such as wheat (bread, pasta, cereals), starch (potatoes, beans, legumes) or fruit. The small exceptions to this are avocados which are a great source of fat (just remember, keep carbs under 20g).

With each week, we're going to focus on the different aspects of the diet, and how they can all help you to reach your best body and health ever.

PREPARING TO START

Before you make any life change, it's important to have a plan. If you try to hit ketosis without planning, you might find that the changes are overwhelming and quit. The thing is, preparing for a major life change is never easy, so how do you do it?

These tips can make your transition much easier and offer better, faster results:

- Choose a start date: Choose a date that you feel like you'll be ready to get started. Mondays are usually best, because it's the beginning of the week. Try to plan for a week or two out, so you can prepare yourself for the changes you'll be making. Take this time to pump yourself up and get going on your lifestyle changes.

- Decide why you want to start the Keto diet: So, why do you really want to get started on the Keto diet? Chances are, you want to lose weight and get rid of that unsightly fat, but there might be other reasons, too. Maybe you don't feel as good as you would like to. Maybe you're feeling unhappy and anxious. It's even possible that you're struggling with some depression. The Keto diet can help. When you know why you're changing the way you eat, you'll be able to keep your focus to see if your changes really work.

- Set some goals: What are you hoping to accomplish with the Keto diet? Do you want to drop a few pants sizes, improve your health, or just get to feeling better? Do you want to work on living a healthier lifestyle? No matter what your goals are, making the changes that come with the Keto diet is going to be much easier when you know what you're working toward.

- Take notes: While this workbook can help, you're also going to want to keep track of each day of your new lifestyle. This helps you to get familiar with your body and gain a solid understanding of what feels good, what doesn't and what offers solid results. So, plan a time each day to take notes of your progress, how you're feeling, what is working and what isn't.

- Determine how long you'll work at your Keto diet: Yes, it's a lifestyle, but let's be real, whenever you make a change like the way you eat, you're going to want to know if there's an end in sight. So, for now, let's decide how long you're going to work at your keto diet. If you give the basic plan a fair shake (I like to say about a month, which is why I offer a four week program), you can begin to make slight changes to fit your lifestyle and keep you enjoying the results you've gained so far.

Once you've taken all these steps to prepare to get started with your Keto diet, it's time to familiarize yourself with more about what makes this type of diet work. I've given you an easy breakdown, but since there is so much information out there, you're going to want to gain as much knowledge as you can.

Remember, knowledge is power, and in this case, the better your understanding of this diet, the more likely it is that you'll be able to stick with your changes for the long-term. I've included some solid resources on the website, so be sure to check them out.

PREPARING TO START KETO

Keto diet start date: _____

Today's date: _____

How am I preparing myself to start the Keto diet? _____

_____

_____

_____

Why do I want to start the Keto diet? _____

_____

_____

_____

What do I hope to make happen with the Keto diet overall? _____

_____

_____

_____

Right now, I'm feeling physically (fill in the blank): _____

_____

I'm feeling mentally (fill in the blank): _____

_____

I'm planning to continue with the Keto diet for at least: _____

WHAT YOU CAN — AND CAN'T — EAT ON THE KETO DIET

As with all diets, there are some foods you really shouldn't eat, and there are some foods you should fill yourself up on. Unfortunately, those gorgeous triple chocolate pecan cookies aren't allowed on the keto diet, either, so have a couple before you start, and get ready to curb your cravings for them forever!

Keto friendly foods:

We will get much more into detail later on about what foods you can really enjoy on this diet, as well as which ones can make a solid difference for your overall health, but for now, here is a list of the foods that are not only allowed, but that you should enjoy.

- Protein. Fish, beef, lamb poultry, and eggs
- Leafy greens. Spinach, kale, romaine lettuce, arugula lettuce
- High fat dairy products. Hard cheeses, high fat cream, high quality butter, and sour cream
- Nuts and seeds. Walnuts, sunflower seeds, pecans, and macadamia nuts
- Olives
- Avocado
- Sweeteners. Monk fruit, stevia, erythritol
- Other healthy fats. Olive oil, coconut oil, high fat salad dressings, and saturated fats

Foods to avoid

While you know those cookies are off the list, you should consider why. In this case, it's not the calories that cause the biggest problem, it's the carbs and sugar. When you're on a keto diet, it's important to try to avoid most types of sugars, because the take the body out of ketosis. This is because sugars are some of the easiest types of energy sources the body can find to digest. So, you'll find that most of the not allowed foods are carbs (which break down into sugar), or sugars themselves.

- Sugar. Avoid honey, maple syrup, agave and all other types of sugars
- Grains. Cereal, corn, rice and wheat are off the table
- Fruits. Avoid bananas, apples, oranges, grapes and other types of sweet tasting fruits
- Tubers. Yams, sweet potatoes and potatoes are all no-go foods
- Bread. Even low carb bread has too many carbs for the keto diet

Understanding processed and prepared foods

If you really want to get the best results with the Keto diet, you're going to want to avoid processed foods whenever possible. However, life gets busy, and meals are often hard to come by. So, be prepared, and read the labels. You'll probably get really good at keeping track of your carbohydrate intake, but for now, remember that the lower, the better.

What about veggies?

You hear a lot about protein and fat when you're on the keto diet. Many of us hear Keto and think, "steak, avocado, and eggs." There is much more that you can enjoy than you might realize. This is where veggies come in.

For most of your meals, you're going to want to include some kind of dark, leafy green. Think spinach, kale, arugula and the like.

Essentially, for your meals, you're looking for a balance of protein, veggies and extra fat. Chicken breast basted in olive oil, broccoli and cheese, is a great example of a keto friendly meal. Or, steak with a knob of butter on top, and a side of spinach that has been sautéed in olive oil is also a solid Keto meal.

Fats and Oils

You know you need to eat fat and oil, but what is considered to be a good choice? Fats seem to go against all we have been trained to consume, so this one might be a bit of a challenge.

So, here's what you need to know. You will want most of your calories to come from fats, and you can even add them to any and all your meals, and even your coffee.

Good fat examples:

- Fatty Fish
- Lard
- Avocados
- Macadamia/Brazil Nuts
- Mayonnaise
- Cocoa Butter
- Coconut Oil
- Macadamia Oil
- Animal Fat (non-hydrogenated)
- Tallow
- Egg Yolks
- Butter/Ghee
- Coconut Butter
- Olive Oil
- Avocado Oil
- MCT Oil

When it comes to protein

Most of us think we know about protein. Eggs. Peanut butter. Meat. But, what are really solid sources of the good stuff?

Examples of optimal protein sources:

- Fish. Preferably eating anything that is caught wild like catfish, cod, flounder, halibut, mackerel, mahi-mahi, salmon, snapper, trout, and tuna. Fattier fish is better.

- Shellfish. Clams, oysters, lobster, crab, scallops, mussels, and squid.

- Whole Eggs. Try to get them free-range from the local market if possible. You can prepare them in many different ways like fried, deviled, boiled, poached, and scrambled.

- Beef. Ground beef, steak, roasts, and stew meat. Stick with fattier cuts where possible. If you can get grass fed, that's a better option.

- Pork. Ground pork, pork loin, pork chops, tenderloin, and ham. Watch out for added sugars and try to stick with fattier cuts.
- Poultry. Chicken, duck, quail, pheasant and other wild game.
- Offal/Organ. Heart, liver, kidney, and tongue. Offal is one of the best sources of vitamins/nutrients.
- Other Meat. Veal, Goat, Lamb, Turkey and other wild game. Stick with fattier cuts where possible.
- Bacon and Sausage. Check labels for anything cured in sugar, or if it contains extra fillers. There are bacons with no sugar added. Check local grocery store
- Nut Butter. Go for natural, unsweetened nuts and try to stick with fattier versions like almond butter and macadamia nut butter. When starting off on the keto diet, I would hold off on nut butters.

Is dairy good or bad?

This is a mixed bag, because some people are sensitive to dairy, but we will talk about that later. If you have a three glass of milk a day habit, this will be tough for you, but you can get your calcium from many other sources, and dairy isn't completely off the table with the Keto diet.

Examples of good dairy sources:

- Heavy whipping cream
- Cream cheese, sour cream, mascarpone, creme fraiche, etc.
- Soft Cheese including mozzarella, brie, blue, Colby, Monterey jack, etc.
- Hard Cheese including aged cheddar, parmesan, feta, swiss, etc.
- Mayonnaise and mayo alternatives that include dairy. Read the labels for any added sugars.

So, even though those three glasses of milk a day might not be a good option (too much sugar), you will probably find a ton of great ways to get your calcium and the protein and healthy fat your body needs.

UNDERSTANDING MACROS

You might have heard of macros and thought that they would be far too complicated to keep track of. While they definitely add a bit of work to your usual eating routine, remember that you're working to pay attention to how your body feels, anyway.

While we won't focus on macros until week two of my program, you're still going to want to have a solid understanding of them, so the transition doesn't feel too complicated. Remember, the goal is to help make things as easy as possible, so you can turn this into your life.

The basic breakdown

One thing to keep in mind is that a good keto diet is high in fat, moderate in protein and very low in carbs. So, the nutrients you take in should break down something like this:

- 75% healthy fats
- 20% protein
- 5% carbohydrates

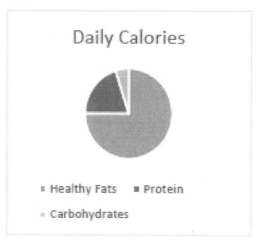

The thing is, figuring percentages can be tough. The main thing you really need to worry about is your carb intake. You should go no higher than 30g a day. This is for an everyday diet. If you're trying to control your sugar and lose weight, you're going to want to stay at about 20g of carbs each day.

When you read a label, that's not a lot, but you'll get used to it and will probably find that there is actually a lot you can eat.

Essential for positive results with keto: Keep carb intake between 20 and 30 grams. ***For best health and weight loss results, stay around 20 grams of carbohydrates each day***

It's also a good idea to keep track of your net carbs and total carbs each day while you're trying to gain weight loss and health results.

If you're confused, don't worry. You'll get the hang of it. For now, you should just remember to eat your protein as you need to, and then add healthy fats to make up the bulk of the remainder of each meal. For our proposes, you're going to keep track of your total carb intake, not the net carbs.

Making it work

When I first started the Keto diet, I found my head was swimming. It seemed like everything had carbs and figuring it all out was so complicated. That's why I am making this workbook and creating several cheat sheets to help you get the best start possible. I also want you to see results and have as easy a time as possible turning this into a lifestyle that you can comfortably enjoy.

For now, pay attention to cutting out things like bread, pasta, pastries and cakes. You should also make it a point to enjoy meals that are high in protein and healthy fats. Scrambled eggs and avocado are favorites of mine, but certainly not your only choices.

WHAT ABOUT THE DREADED "KETO FLU?"

If you've been looking into the keto diet for any amount of time, you've probably heard of the keto flu. It sounds miserable, doesn't it? Why would anyone voluntarily get sick from a diet? It's completely normal and happens for a number of reasons.

The good news is that it's incredibly common, and it only lasts a few days. Plus, I've found some solid ways to help make it better, or even avoid it.

The symptoms include headache, fatigue, cramps, nausea, etc.

Why you get the keto flu

The two primary reasons that people wind up with the keto flu include:

- Keto is a diuretic. You tend to go to the bathroom more to urinate, which attributes to a loss of both electrolytes and water in your body. You can usually help combat this by drinking chicken stock, bone broth, or adding a pinch of salt under your tongue (my personal trick). A non-negotiable trick is increasing your water intake. Mainly, you want to replenish your depleted electrolytes.

- You're in transition mode. Your body is equipped to process a high intake of carbs and a lower intake of fat. Therefore, when you're transitioning to burning mostly fat, your body needs to create enzymes to be able to do this. In the transitional period, the brain may run low on energy which can lead to brain fog, nausea, and headaches.

After increasing water intake, adding salt, and replacing electrolytes, it should relieve most to all symptoms of Keto Flu. *Tip: Pink Himalayan salt works best when combating the keto flu.*

IF YOU'RE READY TO GET STARTED

So, if you're ready to get started, here we go. This is where you get to do some work, but don't worry, it won't be too hard!

Make sure to keep track of your progress, and goals so that you can see just how much progress you're making. The following workbook pages will help you to see what to change, what to keep, and what really works for you.

PULL OUT PAGES

What to look for in Keto Friendly Foods:

- **Fats & Oils.** Try to get your fat from natural sources like meat and nuts. Supplement with saturated and monounsaturated fats like coconut oil, butter, and olive oil.

- **Protein.** Try to stick with organic, pasture-raised and grass-fed meat where possible. Most meats don't have added sugar in them, so they can be consumed in moderate quantity. Remember to keep the protein moderate

- **Vegetables.** Fresh or frozen doesn't matter. Stick with above ground vegetables, leaning toward leafy/green items.

- **Dairy.** Most dairy is fine, but make sure to buy full-fat dairy items. Harder cheeses typically have fewer carbs.

- **Nuts and Seeds.** In moderation, nuts and seeds can be used to create some fantastic textures. Try to use fattier nuts like macadamias and walnuts. Tips: Nuts can be addictive so measure out before consuming.

- **Beverages.** Stay simple and stick to mostly water. You can consume flavored sparkling water with natural flavoring.

What to drink

- **Water.** You can drink still or sparkling water.
- **Bone Broth.** A great source for electrolyte balance
- **Coffee.** Great focus booster
- **Tea.** Has the same effects as coffee, but many don't enjoy tea. Try to stick with black or green.
- **Coconut/Almond milk.** You can use the unsweetened versions in the carton from the store to replace your favorite dairy beverage.
- **Diet soda.** Try to severely reduce or completely stop drinking this. It can lead to sugar cravings and sometimes insulin spikes in the long run.
- **Flavoring.** The small packets that are flavored with sucralose or stevia are fine. You can alternatively add a squeeze of lemon, lime, or orange to your water bottle.
- **Alcohol.** You can choose wine or alcohol, just stay under 20 grams. Tip: Alchohol takes 12 hours to process through the liver so this can delay as weight loss. I would recommend no alcohol for the first month.

WEEK ONE FOOD JOURNAL

The first week of my Mindfulness Keto four-week program will largely involve getting your body into ketosis. This will help your body change the way it gains energy. You're going from depending on the quick energy of sugars and carbs, to the slower, harder to get to fat. When you're in ketosis, you're right where you want to be in terms of fat burning, body sculpting weight loss. In terms of your health, you're likely to find that getting rid of all that sugar is going to boost your overall wellness tremendously.

So, this week, the goal is to keep track of the foods you eat. Be sure to take note of how you prepare your food, too. This will be your guide for foods that work, and foods that don't.

This week my health and wellness goals are: _____
_____
_____

Monday: Breakfast: _____

Lunch: _____

Dinner: _____

Total Carbs: _____

Tuesday: Breakfast: _____

Lunch: _____

Dinner: _____

Total Carbs: _____

Wednesday: Breakfast: _____

Lunch: _____

Dinner: _____

Total Carbs: _____

Thursday: Breakfast: _____

Lunch: _____

Dinner: _____

Total Carbs: _____

Friday: Breakfast: _____

Lunch: _____

Dinner: _____

Total Carbs: _____

Saturday: Breakfast: _____

Lunch: _____

Dinner: _____

Total Carbs: _____

Sunday: Breakfast: _____

Lunch: _____

Dinner: _____

Total Carbs: _____

On Monday I weighed: _____

On Sunday I weighed: _____

The days I felt the best were: _____

What made me feel so good? _____

_____

_____

The days I felt the worst were: _____

What made me feel so bad? _____

_____

_____

_____

_____

Did I reach my health and wellness goals? _____

_____

_____

If not, how close did I come? _____

What can I do differently for week two? _____

_____

_____

_____

WEEK TWO FOOD JOURNAL

For week two, we will start to focus on overall macros. This will give you a much better picture of what you're eating and help you to refine your diet to gain better health and weight loss results. So, be sure to keep track of them. You might be surprised what you just naturally gravitate to when it comes to foods.

Also, now might be a good time to start trying intermittent fasting. ***Be sure to talk to your doctor before trying fasting!*** Start slowly. Make a fairly broad window (like maybe 6 or 8 hours) of eating time to start so you won't feel deprived.

My health and wellness goals for week two are: _____
_____
_____

Monday: Breakfast: _____

Lunch: _____

Dinner: _____

Protein: _____

Carbs: _____

Fat: _____

Fasting hours: _____ Eating hours: _____

Tuesday: Breakfast: _____

Lunch: _____

Dinner: _____

Protein: _____

Carbs: _____

Fat: _____

Fasting hours: _____ Eating hours: _____

Wednesday: Breakfast: _____

Lunch: _____

Dinner: _____

Protein: _____

Carbs: _____

Fat: _____

Fasting hours: _____   Eating hours: _____

Thursday: Breakfast:_____

Lunch: _____

Dinner: _____

Protein: _____

Carbs: _____

Fat: _____

Fasting hours: _____   Eating hours: _____

Friday: Breakfast: _____

Lunch: _____

Dinner: _____

Protein: _____

Carbs: _____

Fat: _____

Fasting hours: _____   Eating hours: _____

Saturday: Breakfast: _____

Lunch: _____

Dinner: _____

Protein: _____

Carbs: _____

Fat: _____

Fasting hours: _____   Eating hours: _____

Sunday: Breakfast: _____

Lunch: _____

Dinner: _____

Protein: _____

Carbs: _____

Fat: _____

Fasting hours: _____   Eating hours: _____

On Monday I weighed: _____

On Sunday I weighed: _____

The days I felt the best were: _____

What made me feel so good? _____

_____

_____

The days I felt the worst were: _____

What made me feel so bad? _____

_____

_____

Did I reach my health and wellness goals? _____

_____

_____

If not, how close did I come? _____

What can I do differently in week three? _____

_____

_____

_____

WEEK THREE FOOD JOURNAL

By now, you should be seeing some improvement in the way you feel. You're probably even getting close to your weight loss goals! Now is the time to keep going and get used to solidifying your new eating habits. You should have found some keto food favorites, and you should have a good idea of what's going to work for you.

Have you started modifying your favorite recipes to meet your individual keto needs? Now is the time to get started!

For instance, broccoli cheese and rice soup can be a favorite. Add some chicken, and you have a solid source of protein, but with all that rice, you're adding a ton of carbs, too. You can still enjoy broccoli cheese soup with rice, as long as it's cauliflower rice!

This week my health and wellness goals are: _____
_____
_____

Monday: Breakfast: _____

Lunch: _____

Dinner: _____

Protein: _____

Carbs: _____

Fat: _____

Fasting hours: _____ Eating hours: _____

Tuesday: Breakfast: _____

Lunch: _____

Dinner: _____

Protein: _____

Carbs: _____

Fat: _____

Fasting hours: _____ Eating hours: _____

Wednesday: Breakfast: _____

Lunch: _____

Dinner: _____

Protein: _____

Carbs: _____

Fat: _____

Fasting hours: _____   Eating hours: _____

Thursday: Breakfast: _____

Lunch: _____

Dinner: _____

Protein: _____

Carbs: _____

Fat: _____

Fasting hours: _____   Eating hours: _____

Friday: Breakfast: _____

Lunch: _____

Dinner: _____

Protein: _____

Carbs: _____

Fat: _____

Fasting hours: _____   Eating hours: _____

Saturday: Breakfast: _____

Lunch: _____

Dinner: _____

Protein: _____

Carbs: _____

Fat: _____

Fasting hours: _____   Eating hours: _____

Sunday: Breakfast: _____

Lunch: _____

Dinner: _____

Protein: _____

Carbs: _____

Fat: _____

Fasting hours: _____   Eating hours: _____

On Monday I weighed: _____

On Sunday I weighed: _____

The days I felt the best were: _____

What made me feel so good? _____

_____

_____

The days I felt the worst were: _____

What made me feel so bad? _____

_____

_____

The days I felt worse were: _____

Why did I feel so bad? _____

_____

_____

Did I reach my health and wellness goals? _____

If not, how close did I come? What could I do differently for week four? _____

_____

_____

What are some ways I can modify my favorite foods? _____

_____

_____

_____

WEEK FOUR FOOD JOURNAL

Here you are!!! Week four!!! This is the point where you're going to feel like you've traveled a thousand miles. If you're working toward losing weight, you're probably getting close to seeing some serious results. Now, you might not be all the way there, but don't lose heart. Just keep going with the lifestyle and you will reach your goals.

While you might not have hit a plateau just yet, you're probably close to getting there. So, if you're still on the way to reaching your goals, you might also be feeling a bit frustrated. Don't be. I've got cheat sheets that will help you keep going strong. So, let's do this last week!

Oh, and now is a good time to consider whether you're going to keep going with the Keto diet. Even if you choose to use it to maintain your recent health changes, you might find by now that you're feeling pretty amazing. So, maybe sticking with it is a good idea after all!

My health and wellness goals for week four are: _____

_____

_____

Monday: Breakfast: _____

Lunch: _____

Dinner: _____

Protein: _____

Carbs: _____

Fat: _____

Fasting hours: _____ Eating hours: _____

Tuesday: Breakfast: _____

Lunch: _____

Dinner: _____

Protein: _____

Carbs: _____

Fat: _____

Fasting hours: _____ Eating hours: _____

Wednesday: Breakfast: _____

Lunch: _____

Dinner: _____

Protein: _____

Carbs: _____

Fat: _____

Fasting hours: _____   Eating hours: _____

Thursday: Breakfast: _____

Lunch: _____

Dinner: _____

Protein: _____

Carbs: _____

Fat: _____

Fasting hours: _____   Eating hours: _____

Friday: Breakfast: _____

Lunch: _____

Dinner: _____

Protein: _____

Carbs: _____

Fat: _____

Fasting hours: _____   Eating hours: _____

Saturday: Breakfast: _____

Lunch: _____

Dinner: _____

Protein: _____

Carbs: _____

Fat: _____

Fasting hours: _____   Eating hours: _____

Sunday: Breakfast: _____

Lunch: _____

Dinner: _____

Protein: _____

Carbs: _____

Fat: _____

Fasting hours: _____ Eating hours: _____

On Monday I weighed: _____

On Sunday I weighed: _____

The days I felt the best were: _____

What made me feel so good? _____

_____

_____

The days I felt the worst were: _____

What made me feel so bad? _____

_____

_____

The days I felt worse were: _____

Why did I feel so bad? _____

_____

_____

Did I reach my health and wellness goals? _____

If not, how close did I come? What could I do differently going forward?_____

_____

_____

Now is the time to offer you a great big *CONGRATULATIONS!!!* You finished your four-week keto plan!

If you're going to keep going, now is the time to decide how much weight you want to lose, or what health goals you want to reach. Remember, keto isn't just to help you look great. It's to help you get healthy in so many ways.

From diabetes, to blood pressure, to depression and fatigue, I firmly believe that the Keto diet can absolutely change your life. So, maybe keep going for a while and see how it goes. After all, all you have to lose is extra fat, but you have all to gain!

Made in the USA
Columbia, SC
08 July 2024

38304900R10017